CREATED BY

Ashley Loren

originally posted on
"A Glass Kingdom" blog and instagram
@a_glass_kingdom

Follow "A Glass Kingdom" on Instagram for more
awesome content and head over to
agkblog.wixsite.com/a-glass-kingdom
(or scan the QR code below with your phone's
camera) to visit and subscribe.

Anxiety

MENTAL HEALTH SERIES

Volume 1

UP NEXT

Anxiety II: For Men

SOON TO FOLLOW

Depression

Trauma

Chronic Illness

Grief

Printed in the United States of America.

First printing, 2022

www.agkblog.wixsite.com/a-glass-kingdom

INTRODUCTION

These days, everybody seems to have an opinion about how to deal with anxiety. "Think positive" they say. "Try some yoga and deep breathing", "Probiotics for the win!" but nothing really works or lasts. Anxiety plagues us; fear overwhelms us, and the world grows darker and shadier by the minute. Though bookshelves are overcrowded with advice, curative methods and thoughts on how to find and maintain peace in this crazy world, only a select few people seem to genuinely possess peace.

Why is that?

This was the question I was faced with a couple of years ago when I started the layout of what would become this journal. I had looked everywhere for peace; everywhere for resources that could handle the severity and rawness of my anxious thoughts while drawing me closer to God at the same time. But I couldn't find anything that worked long-term. Those heavy-weights and burdens always found their way back to me like a chronic cough no one really knew how to get rid of, and if you're holding this book, you can probably relate. Maybe you've prayed a million prayers and asked God to make it go away but it's still here. Maybe you've torn through the pages of your Bible looking for answers, feeling like all you actually found were nice anecdotes. Maybe you've had to start taking medication for anxiety and along with the side effects came this voice that said, "you're a Christian, you shouldn't need medication", "you've got God, you shouldn't need therapy". Whatever situation you find yourself in with anxiety, let me encourage you with this simple yet hard-won truth:

PEACE IS REAL.

Not only is it real but it's yours; it belongs to you. Peace is your inheritance as a child of God. The second Jesus moved into your heart; the prince of peace became your companion; your source; your literal soulmate. You were never meant to be a creature of burden. The weight you've been carrying wasn't meant for your shoulders and the reason your spirit feels broken is because it knows that. Your spirit knows that you're functioning outside of how God intended you to function; that you are taking on battles and wars you were never meant to fight, especially not alone. But even here, even where you feel hopeless and stuck, rest assured. No matter how impossible or chaotic things seem, peace is not beyond you're reach because you are never beyond His.

The reason every other solution falls devastatingly short is because true healing can only be found with the true healer. Nothing can force anxiety out of your life and out of your mind better than the presence of God. His presence leaves no room for fear to dwell, His word annihilates anxiety where it stands and that's what this journal/journey is all about. Inviting God into your process and into your brokenness. Creating a habit of laying your burdens down at His feet. Establishing a pattern of transparency in your life and in your relationship with God, where you learn how to surrender to Him, even when things are messy and ugly. Even when YOU are messy and ugly.

With that said, let me just clarify, what you're holding in your hands right now is nothing more than a tool. Beautifully designed and God-driven, it's true. However, the power behind this tool rests solely between you and God and what you make of this space.

So, what will you make of it?

SCAN & LISTEN
to the songs of the day on spotify

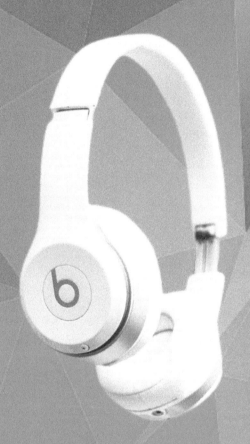

HOW TO SCAN

Open your Spotify app and click the search icon. You should have the browse/search page open
that has recommendations and genres of music displayed. At the top right corner you'll see a
camera icon. Click it and "allow" it permission to use your camera. Then simply point your
camera at the graphic barcode above and it will take you to the playlist.

Worry page intentions.

What is a 'worry page'?

It's a place for you to purge the anxious thoughts that you struggle with throughout the day.
It's a place to lay down your burdens and give your worries over to God. A place to let it all out,
no judgement, no limits, nobody else but you and God.

Why do I need it?

Sometimes we need a physical reminder and representation of surrender to help us live it out.
And sometimes, it's hard to sort through an anxious mind;
to grab ahold of our faith using just our mental stamina.
This worry time allows us the space to vent and be honest about things we can't say or don't
know how to say to others. And these pages give us a physical place to put our burdens.

What do I do?

Everyday, take a second to write down all of the anxieties and worries clouding your mind.
Whatever you're struggling with, whatever is bothering you.
Get it all out on the page and surrender it to God.
When you're done, you can turn the page and start a fresh new day
or you can do something symbolic with those worries.
You could scribble over all your fears with a pen and cross them out.
You could write a positive declaration over the whole page with a marker or cut the page out
(very carefully because the paper is not perforated) and crumble it in your fist; tear it to
shreds and then throw your worries in the trash where they belong.
I've even noticed that sometimes, as I'm writing my worries down, God will start speaking to me
about them, so I'll take a different colored pen and write whatever He's sharing with me next to
the worry He's referencing. But this is your journal, so, it's completely up to you.

My hope is that by the end of this book you'll run out of worries to write down and the last few
of these pages will remain empty. Not because everything has suddenly become perfect and you
have no more worries but because you've learned how to put them where they belong; how to
put them in the hands of the one who loves you and cares for you the most.
But if you need each and every page cause your heart is just that heavy, they're here for you.
God is here for you; with you in every second of your surrender and He will continue to help you
lay down those burdens even as you run out of journal. I pray that through these pages and
these 31 days of scripture God will help you practice exchanging your anxiety for His peace
because you have access; you have the option and peace belongs to you, more than anxiety
could ever hope to. Amen?

DAY 1

JOHN 14:27

Song of the day
HERE I AM
JORDAN MAY

ANXIETY IS ALWAYS TELLING US HOW THINGS COULD GO WRONG.
TODAY, PICK A FEW RECURRING ANXIETIES AND WRITE THEM DOWN IN
THE LEFT COLUMN. IN THE RIGHT COLUMN, REFRAME THOSE THOUGHTS
BY WRITING DOWN THE WAYS THOSE THINGS COULD GO RIGHT

Worry page

God, here I lay my burdens down at your feet.
What's on this page no longer belongs to me,
it's in your hands.

Worry page

God, here I lay my burdens down at your feet.
What's on this page no longer belongs to me,
it's in your hands.

DAY 2

PHILIPPIANS 4:4-7

WHAT ARE 3 THINGS YOU ARE GRATEFUL FOR TODAY?

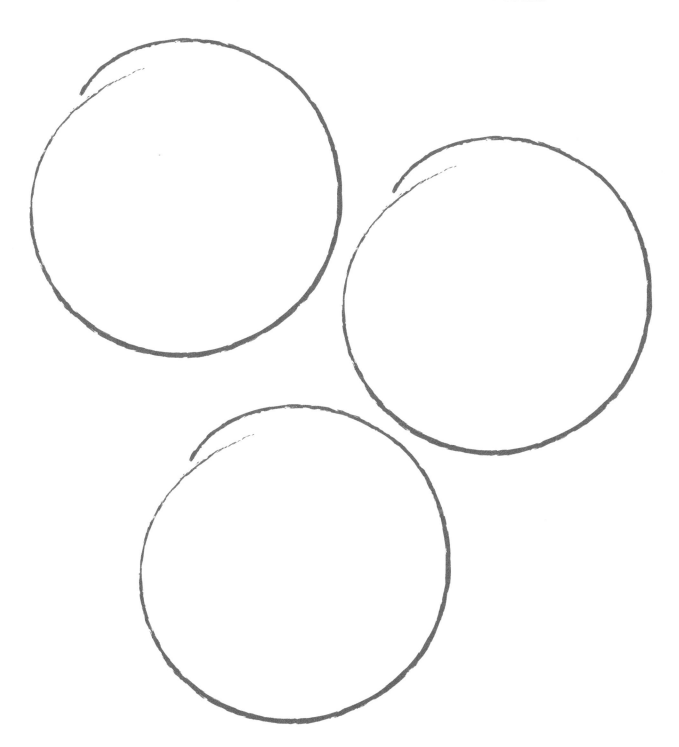

DAY 3

PSALM 121:1-8

DATE: / /

WHEN YOU FEEL ANXIOUS OR OVERWHELMED, WHAT DO YOU ESCAPE TO? IS IT A HOBBY, THE TV, A SIN, ETC.?

_____

WHAT DO YOU THINK YOU'RE SEARCHING FOR IN THE PLACES YOU ESCAPE TO?

_____
_____
_____
_____
_____
_____
_____
_____
_____
_____
_____
_____
_____
_____
_____
_____

Worry page

God, here I lay my burdens down at your feet.
What's on this page no longer belongs to me,
it's in your hands.

Worry page

God, here I lay my burdens down at your feet.
What's on this page no longer belongs to me,
it's in your hands.

DAY 4

ISAIAH 26:3-4

DATE: / /

Song of the day

FOREVER AMEN
STEFFANY GRETZINGER

IF YOU'RE GOOD AT WORRYING, YOU'LL BE GREAT AT WORSHIP; IT'S JUST
THE SAME IMAGINATION WITH A DIFFERENT FOCUS.
SO, WHAT ARE SOME THINGS ABOUT GOD'S CHARACTER (WHO HE IS)
THAT YOU LOVE AND APPRECIATE? AND WHY DO THOSE STAND OUT?

DAY 5

MATTHEW 11:28-30

Song of the day
ANXIOUS
SARAH REEVES

IF YOU COULD LIVE A LIFE FREE OF ANXIETY WHO WOULD YOU BE?
WHAT COULD YOU ACCOMPLISH IF YOU WERE ABLE TO LIVE IN FULL
CONFIDENCE AND PEACE?

_____

_____

_____

_____

_____

_____

_____

_____

_____

_____

_____

_____

_____

_____

_____

Worry page

God, here I lay my burdens down at your feet.
What's on this page no longer belongs to me,
it's in your hands.

Worry page

God, here I lay my burdens down at your feet.
What's on this page no longer belongs to me,
it's in your hands.

DAY 6

PSALM 18:1-19

WRITE DOWN 3 WAYS GOD HAS BLESSED YOU THIS YEAR?

DAY 7

MATTHEW 6:31-34

WHAT EXACTLY HAS WORRY ACCOMPLISHED FOR YOU LATELY? REALLY THINK ABOUT IT, DID IT SAVE YOU FROM PAIN, DID IT PREPARE YOU? DID IT GET THE BILLS PAID OR MAKE ANYTHING BETTER? WHAT ABOUT FAITH? WHAT HAS FAITH DONE FOR YOU LATELY?

WORRY

_____
_____
_____
_____
_____
_____
_____

FAITH

_____
_____
_____
_____
_____
_____

Worry page

God, here I lay my burdens down at your feet.
What's on this page no longer belongs to me,
it's in your hands.

Worry page

God, here I lay my burdens down at your feet.
What's on this page no longer belongs to me,
it's in your hands.

DAY 8

JOHN 16:33

IF YOUR ANXIETY WAS SOMEONE YOU COULD SPEAK TO, WHAT WOULD YOU SAY TO IT?

DAY 9

ISAIAH 41:10

IN WHAT WAYS DO YOU NEED GOD TO...

STRENGTHEN YOU

_____

_____

_____

_____

HELP YOU

_____

_____

_____

_____

HOLD YOU UP

_____

_____

_____

_____

Worry page

God, here I lay my burdens down at your feet.
What's on this page no longer belongs to me,
it's in your hands.

Worry page

God, here I lay my burdens down at your feet.
What's on this page no longer belongs to me,
it's in your hands.

DAY 10

PSALM 27

Song of the day
SEE ME THROUGH IT
BRANDON HEATH

I FEEL THE MOST CONFIDENT WHEN...

DAY 11

MATTHEW 6:26-29

Song of the day
BIRDS
ANNA GOLDEN

SOME EXAMPLES OF MY FEARS BEING PROVED WRONG ARE...

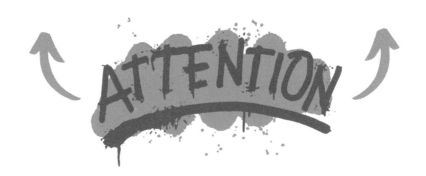

Worry page

God, here I lay my burdens down at your feet.
What's on this page no longer belongs to me,
it's in your hands.

Worry page

God, here I lay my burdens down at your feet.
What's on this page no longer belongs to me,
it's in your hands.

DAY 12

ROMANS 8:26-27

WHAT SITUATIONS IN YOUR LIFE LEAVE YOU FEELING STRESSED OUT, WEAK OR POWERLESS? LIST THEM BELOW AND READ TODAY'S SCRIPTURE OVER AGAIN WHEN YOU'RE DONE WRITING.

DAY 13

PSALM 23:1-4

WHAT IS 1 THING YOU ARE LOOKING FORWARD TO IN THE COMING DAYS, WEEKS OR MONTHS?

Worry page

God, here I lay my burdens down at your feet.
What's on this page no longer belongs to me,
it's in your hands.

Worry page

God, here I lay my burdens down at your feet.
What's on this page no longer belongs to me,
it's in your hands.

DAY 14

ROMANS 8:15-17

IF YOU COULD SPEAK TO SOMEONE ELSE WHO'S BEEN STRUGGLING IN THE SAME AREAS YOU'VE BEEN STRUGGLING, WHAT WOULD YOU WANT TO TELL THEM? TODAY, WRITE AN ENCOURAGING MESSAGE BELOW TO SOMEONE ELSE STRUGGLING WITH ANXIETY

To my fellow plant growing through concrete,

_____

_____

_____

_____

_____

_____

_____

_____

_____

_____

_____

_____

DAY 15

JOHN 17:6-26

DID YOU KNOW THAT JESUS PRAYED OVER YOU? AS YOU REFLECT ON TODAY'S VERSE AND JESUS'S PRAYER, REWRITE WHAT YOU WROTE DOWN YESTERDAY, EXCEPT THIS TIME, WRITE IT TO YOURSELF.

Dear me,

_____

_____

_____

_____

_____

_____

_____

_____

_____

_____

_____

_____

_____

Day 15 JOHN 17:6-26

Worry page

God, here I lay my burdens down at your feet.
What's on this page no longer belongs to me,
it's in your hands.

Worry page

God, here I lay my burdens down at your feet.
What's on this page no longer belongs to me,
it's in your hands.

DAY 16

1 PETER 5:6-7

I AM PROUD OF MYSELF BECAUSE...

_____

_____

_____

_____

_____

_____

_____

_____

_____

_____

_____

_____

_____

_____

_____

DAY 17

JOHN 10:27-28

FIND A SCRIPTURE THAT YOU CAN APPLY TO YOUR ANXIETY, SOMETHING MEANINGFUL TO YOU AND WRITE IT BELOW. MEMORIZE IT AND REPEAT IT SO THAT WHEN YOU FEEL ANXIOUS TODAY OR ANYTIME THIS WEEK, YOU CAN RECITE THAT SCRIPTURE OVER AND OVER AGAIN UNTIL YOU FEEL SATISFIED.

Worry page

God, here I lay my burdens down at your feet.
What's on this page no longer belongs to me,
it's in your hands.

Worry page

God, here I lay my burdens down at your feet.
What's on this page no longer belongs to me,
it's in your hands.

DAY 18

2 CORINTHIANS 4:16-18

Song of the day
CAPTURED
ISLA VISTA WORSHIP,
MARK BARLOW

WHO DOES YOUR ANXIETY SAY GOD IS? WHEN YOU'RE ANXIOUS, WHAT VERSION OF GOD DOES YOUR MIND CREATE?
(A DISTANT GOD OR AN UNLOVING DISCIPLINARIAN? A GOD TOO HOLY TO LOWER HIMSELF WITH YOU? A NON-EXISTENT GOD?)

_____

_____

_____

_____

_____

_____

_____

_____

_____

_____

_____

_____

_____

_____

DAY 19

2 TIMOTHY 1:7

Song of the day
PEACE BE STILL
HOPE DARST

ANXIETY IS NOT YOUR IDENTITY; IT IS AN ATTACK ON IT.
SO, WHEN YOU FEEL ANXIOUS, WHAT INSECURITIES OR THOUGHTS
ABOUT YOURSELF DO YOU NOTICE ARE MOST PREVALENT?

Worry page

God, here I lay my burdens down at your feet.
What's on this page no longer belongs to me,
it's in your hands.

Worry page

God, here I lay my burdens down at your feet.
What's on this page no longer belongs to me,
it's in your hands.

DAY 20

PSALM 73:25-26

WHAT DOES IT MEAN TO KNOW THAT GOD, THE CREATOR OF EVERYTHING, IS THE STRENGTH OF YOUR HEART? TO KNOW THAT YOU HAVE AN ETERNAL SOURCE THAT NEVER RUNS OUT KEEPING YOUR HEART BEATING?

_____

_____

_____

_____

_____

_____

_____

_____

_____

_____

_____

_____

_____

DAY 21

PSALM 143:7-10

Song of the day
CLOSE
ROY TOSH
FEAT. EVAN & ERIS

TODAY, TAKE ALL THE SPACE YOU NEED AND WRITE A MESSAGE TO GOD.
JUST LIKE THE PSALMIST, POUR OUT ALL OF YOUR DOUBTS, QUESTIONS, HOPES AND
FEARS ONTO THIS PAPER. TELL GOD EVERYTHING, EVEN IF YOU THINK HE WON'T
LIKE IT, EVEN IF YOU THINK IT WILL MAKE HIM ANGRY. I'M CHALLENGING YOU TO
TELL HIM THE HARD THINGS, THE THINGS YOU THINK DISQUALIFY YOU AND THE
THINGS YOU WOULDN'T DARE TELL ANOTHER SOUL.
IF YOU DON'T WANT TO WRITE IT DOWN, THAT'S OKAY, FIND A QUIET
UNINTERRUPTED SPACE AND START TALKING, LET IT ALL COME INTO THE LIGHT.

God,

_____

_____

_____

_____

_____

_____

_____

_____

_____

_____

_____

_____

_____

Day 21 PSALM 143:7-10

Day 21 PSALM 143:7-10

Worry page

God, here I lay my burdens down at your feet.
What's on this page no longer belongs to me,
it's in your hands.

Worry page

God, here I lay my burdens down at your feet.
What's on this page no longer belongs to me,
it's in your hands.

DAY 22

PSALM 95:6-7

WRITE OUT THE LYRICS TO YOUR FAVORITE WORSHIP SONG BELOW.

my favorite worship song is _____
and it goes like this...

DAY 23

PSALM 145:17-19

WHAT PRAYERS HAVE YOU SEEN ANSWERED? MAYBE IT WAS SOMETHING YOU PRAYED FOR OR SOMETHING SOMEONE ELSE PRAYED FOR.
REMIND YOURSELF GOD STILL ANSWERS PRAYERS BY WRITING DOWN THE EVIDENCE OF HIS FAITHFULNESS THAT YOU'VE SEEN AND HEARD.

Worry page

God, here I lay my burdens down at your feet.
What's on this page no longer belongs to me,
it's in your hands.

Worry page

God, here I lay my burdens down at your feet.
What's on this page no longer belongs to me,
it's in your hands.

DAY 24
PROVERBS 3:5-6

IF YOU COULD TELL SOMEONE IN YOUR LIFE SOMETHING WITHOUT JUDGEMENT AND WITHOUT THEM GETTING UPSET OR HURT, WHO WOULD YOU WANT TO TALK TO AND WHAT WOULD YOU SAY TO THEM?

I would speak to

AND SAY...

_____

_____

_____

_____

_____

_____

_____

_____

_____

_____

_____

_____

_____

_____

_____

_____

DAY 25

ROMANS 8:38-39

Song of the day
LOVED
FRESH LIFE WORSHIP

WHICH OF THESE EMOTIONS DO YOU FIND HARDEST TO ACCEPT?
WHY DO YOU THINK THAT IS?

Happiness

Peace

Love

Compassion

Hope

Generosity

_____

_____

_____

_____

_____

_____

_____

_____

_____

_____

Worry page

God, here I lay my burdens down at your feet.
What's on this page no longer belongs to me,
it's in your hands.

Worry page

God, here I lay my burdens down at your feet.
What's on this page no longer belongs to me,
it's in your hands.

DAY 26

HEBREWS 4:16

WHAT DO YOU NEED TO FORGIVE YOURSELF FOR TODAY?

_____

_____

_____

_____

_____

_____

_____

_____

_____

_____

_____

_____

_____

_____

DAY 27

ROMANS 8:28

Song of the day
SYMPHONY
SWITCH
FEAT. DILLON CHASE

HAVE YOU EVER DONE SOMETHING YOU REGRET? IF YOU COULD GO BACK TO THAT TIME, WHAT WOULD YOU DO DIFFERENTLY (IF ANYTHING)? HOW CAN YOU APPLY THE LESSON FROM THAT EXPERIENCE TO YOUR LIFE TODAY?

_____
_____
_____
_____
_____
_____
_____
_____
_____
_____
_____
_____
_____
_____

Worry page

God, here I lay my burdens down at your feet.
What's on this page no longer belongs to me,
it's in your hands.

Worry page

God, here I lay my burdens down at your feet.
What's on this page no longer belongs to me,
it's in your hands.

DAY 28

PSALM 34:4-10

Song of the day
LIFE IS GOOD
COURTNIE RAMIREZ
FEAT. APOLLO LTD

WRITE DOWN 1 POSITIVE WORD TO DESCRIBE YOURSELF.
WHY DID YOU CHOOSE THAT SPECIFIC WORD?
HOW CAN YOU HOLD ONTO THAT IDENTITY MARKER IN THE MIDST OF ANXIETY?

HELLO
my name is

DAY 29

ISAIAH 54:10

Song of the day
LOVE (REMIX)
WE ARE MESSENGERS
FEAT. MALI MUSIC

WHAT ARE SOME OF THE EXPECTATIONS WEIGHING YOU DOWN? THEY COULD BE THINGS OTHER PEOPLE EXPECT OF YOU, THINGS YOUR JOB EXPECTS OF YOU, THINGS YOU EXPECT OF YOURSELF, ETC.

_____

_____

_____

_____

_____

_____

_____

_____

_____

_____

_____

HOW CAN YOU PRACTICE SOME SELF-CARE TODAY?

_____

Worry page

God, here I lay my burdens down at your feet.
What's on this page no longer belongs to me,
it's in your hands.

Worry page

God, here I lay my burdens down at your feet.
What's on this page no longer belongs to me,
it's in your hands.

DAY 30

COLOSSIANS 1:9-13

MAKE A LIST OF 5 THINGS THAT INSPIRE AND MOTIVATE YOU TO KEEP GOING

DAY 31

PSALM 125:1-2

Song of the day
STARTING NOW
DAVID DUNN

WHAT YOU BELIEVE ABOUT YOURSELF MATTERS MORE THAN WHAT ANXIETY
TELLS YOU ABOUT YOURSELF. SO, WHO DO YOU SAY YOU ARE? FORGET THE
LABELS OTHERS HAVE BURDENED YOU WITH,
FORGET THE PAST, WHO ARE YOU TODAY?
RIGHT HERE AND RIGHT NOW, WHO DO YOU SAY YOU ARE?

I am

I am

I am

I am

I am

I am

Worry page

God, here I lay my burdens down at your feet.
What's on this page no longer belongs to me,
it's in your hands.

Let me pray for you

LORD, I COME BEFORE YOU TODAY WITH A BURDEN ON MY HEART FOR THE PERSON HOLDING THIS JOURNAL IN THEIR HANDS. LORD, YOU KNOW THEIR NAME, THEIR STRUGGLE AND THE BATTLES THEY'VE BEEN FACING LATELY. YOU'VE HEARD THEIR CRIES WHEN THEY WERE TOO SILENT FOR OTHERS TO HEAR AND I KNOW YOUR HEART BREAKS FOR WHAT BREAKS THEIRS. GOD, COME ALONGSIDE YOUR CHILD RIGHT NOW AND WRAP YOUR ARMS AROUND THEM, LET YOUR PRESENCE BE KNOWN IN THE PLACE WHERE THEY ARE RESTING RIGHT NOW. STILL THEIR SOUL AND QUIET THEIR MIND WITH YOUR WORDS OF LOVE AND PEACE.

STRENGTHEN THEIR HEART LORD, AND IN THE PLACES WHERE THEY FEEL WEAK AND OUT OF CONTROL, LIFT THEM UP GOD, CARRY THEM THROUGH THE STORM. HOLD THEM CLOSE TO YOUR CHEST AND LIFT UP THEIR CHIN; HELP THEM TO BRAVELY FACE THE DAYS AHEAD KNOWING YOU GO OUT IN FRONT OF THEM, THE LION OF JUDAH PREPARING THE WAY FOR YOUR LITTLE LAMB. REMIND THEM OF YOUR PLANS FOR THEM, PLANS TO GIVE THEM A FUTURE AND A HOPE. PLANS NOT TO HARM THEM BUT TO RESTORE, REDEEM, HEAL AND UPLIFT THEM GOD. OPEN THEIR EYES WIDER TO SEE THE PURPOSE YOU HAVE INSTILLED WITHIN THEM AND HELP THEM TO WALK FORWARD WITH FULL CONFIDENCE IN THE DOORS YOU WILL OPEN AND THE PATHS YOU HAVE PAVED.

REMIND THEM LORD THAT YOU ARE A FATHER ABOVE ALL, AND NOTHING GOING ON IN THE HEART OF YOUR CHILD IS TOO MUCH FOR YOU TO HANDLE. REMIND THEM THAT YOU HEAR THEIR CRIES, THAT THEY ARE NOT FORGOTTEN OR UNLOVED OR UNSEEN IN THIS SEASON.

SHOW THEM WHO YOU TRULY ARE FOR THEM IN THEIR SUFFERING. THE GOD WHO IS NEAR TO THE BROKENHEARTED; THE GOD WHO LAYS BESIDE THEM WHEN THEY CAN'T GET OUT OF BED; THE GOD WHO WAGES WARS AGAINST EVIL AND DARKNESS IN THE PURSUIT OF JUSTICE FOR EVERY TEAR THEY'VE CRIED; THE GOD WHO ALWAYS WINS; THEIR CHAMPION.

LET YOUR PEACE COMPLETELY ENCOMPASS THEM. GIVE THEM SWEET DREAMS AND VISIONS OF THE PLANS YOU HAVE FOR THEIR LIFE. AND WHEN ANXIETY TRIES TO RISE UP AGAINST THEM, MINISTER TO THEM THROUGH THESE PAGES AND PRACTICES AS YOU HAVE MINISTERED TO ME. LIGHT UP THE SHADOWS IN THEIR MIND WITH YOUR GLORIOUS LIGHT. LET YOUR WORD COME TO THE FOREFRONT OF THEIR MIND AND AS THEY CONFESS IT OVER THEMSELVES, THANK YOU GOD THAT ANXIETY AND FEAR WOULD FLEE IN YOUR PRESENCE. THAT SHAME AND GUILT WOULD RUN FOR THE HILLS CAUSE YOUR PRESENCE SURROUNDS THEM; AND DARKNESS MUST FLEE AT THE SOUND OF YOUR FOOTSTEPS CIRCLING YOUR CHILD. AS THEY SPEAK YOUR WORD OVER THEMSELVES LORD, SET THEM ON FIRE WITH THE TRUTH THEY HOLD, WITH THE POWER THEY CARRY. ERASE ANY OTHER NEGATIVE PRESENCE IN THEIR LIFE AND DON'T LET THEM FORGET WHO THEY ARE. DON'T LET THEM FORGET THAT THEY ARE THE CHILD OF THE STAR-BREATHER AND THAT THEY HAVE AUTHORITY TO SPEAK LIFE OVER THEMSELVES AND OTHERS, TO EXIST IN PEACE AND WALK WITH CONFIDENCE. LORD, I PRAY THAT IN THEIR DAILY LIFE YOU WOULD DO THE HEAVY LIFTING AND THAT YOU WOULD HELP THEM SURRENDER THE BURDENS OF THEIR ANXIOUS HEART TO YOU. LET THEM KNOW THEY ARE SEEN IN THE SHADOWS AND THEY ARE LOVED IN THE DARKNESS.

THANK YOU FOR LEADING THEM HERE, EVEN IF IT WAS JUST FOR THIS PRAYER LORD. AND THANK YOU FOR YOUR KINGDOM WORK IN ME AND IN THE PERSON HOLDING THIS JOURNAL. THANK YOU FOR THEIR LIFE AND THE IMPACT THEY ARE GOING TO MAKE IN THIS WORLD. ANOINT THEM WITH BLESSING LORD, ANOINT THEM WITH YOUR PEACE, FILL THEM WITH HOPE, SOAK THEM WITH JOY AND WATCH OVER THEM IN THEIR COMING AND GOING LIKE THE FIERCE PROTECTOR AND LOVING FATHER I KNOW YOU TO BE.

IN JESUS PRECIOUS NAME, AMEN (SO IT WILL BE)

Ashley Loren

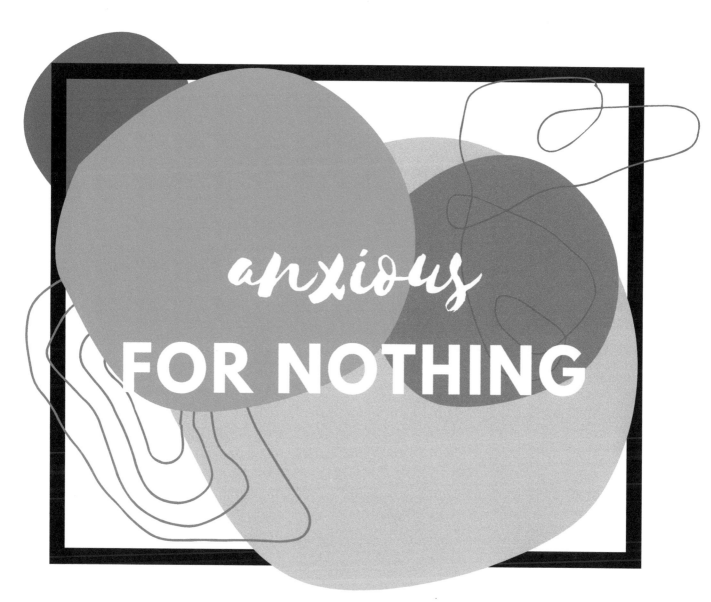

anxious
FOR NOTHING

@a_glass_kingdom

Worry page

God, here I lay my burdens down at your feet.
What's on this page no longer belongs to me,
it's in your hands.

Worry page

God, here I lay my burdens down at your feet.
What's on this page no longer belongs to me,
it's in your hands.

Worry page

God, here I lay my burdens down at your feet.
What's on this page no longer belongs to me,
it's in your hands.

Worry page

God, here I lay my burdens down at your feet.
What's on this page no longer belongs to me,
it's in your hands.

Worry page

God, here I lay my burdens down at your feet.
What's on this page no longer belongs to me,
it's in your hands.

Worry page

God, here I lay my burdens down at your feet.
What's on this page no longer belongs to me,
it's in your hands.

No thought left behind...

No thought left behind...

No thought left behind...

No thought left behind...

No thought left behind...

No thought left behind...

The Method for the Madness

Thanksgiving / Worship *(Philippians 4:6-7)* taking the focus off of what has gone wrong and establishing a new pattern, focusing on what has gone right; seeing the good all around you because there is good all around you. Keeping the good in front of you so you never forget that God has shown Himself faithful

Truth *(Philippians 4:8-9)* Truth is the only thing that has the power to annihilate lies. Rebuking a lie pushes it away for a bit but truth destroys it at the root so, it completely loses its power. Truth is your weapon, your sword. A shield will protect you, but it can't disarm and destroy your enemy like truth. You need to know your truth (an honest assessment of where you're at and why you're there), God's truth (who you are and what has been accomplished for you, so you don't have to stay where you are) and the prevailing truth (what God's truth does with your truth).

Faith *(2 Corinthians 5:7; Hebrews 11:1)* The power to call things that aren't as though they were, to trust God with expectation knowing He is faithful to keep His promises. The authority to speak life over yourself and remain anchored in the storm. To look forward and not back. Even if all you've got is mustard seed sized faith, it's enough

Grace *(2 Corinthians 12:9; Colossians 3:12-15)* Abundant grace for yourself and others enables you to walk forward courageously. It's also the foundation of understanding your identity. Who you are in Christ, is who you are with sufficient grace, that's your truth. Knowing your identity because of grace; knowing who other people are and who they can be because of grace, strengthens you in your fight. Don't let your enemy be the only person on the battlefield that knows who you are; that knows you are more than your sins. Your enemy only reminds you of your sins so you'll never think to look past them and discover who you are on the other side of grace.

Trust *(Isaiah 40:31)* The combination of faith and truth. The utter determination to believe that God is who He says He is and will do what He said He would do. Not leaning on your own understanding or your own assessment of your circumstances. Believing with confident hope that the God of Abraham, Esther, David, Peter and Paul is just as miraculous and faithful to you, as He was to all of them. That His character is shown in His word, and He gave that word to you, not only so you would know who He is, but so you can hold Him to it and take Him at His word.

word, worship, prayer

Anxiety Flow chart

Today I am feeling...

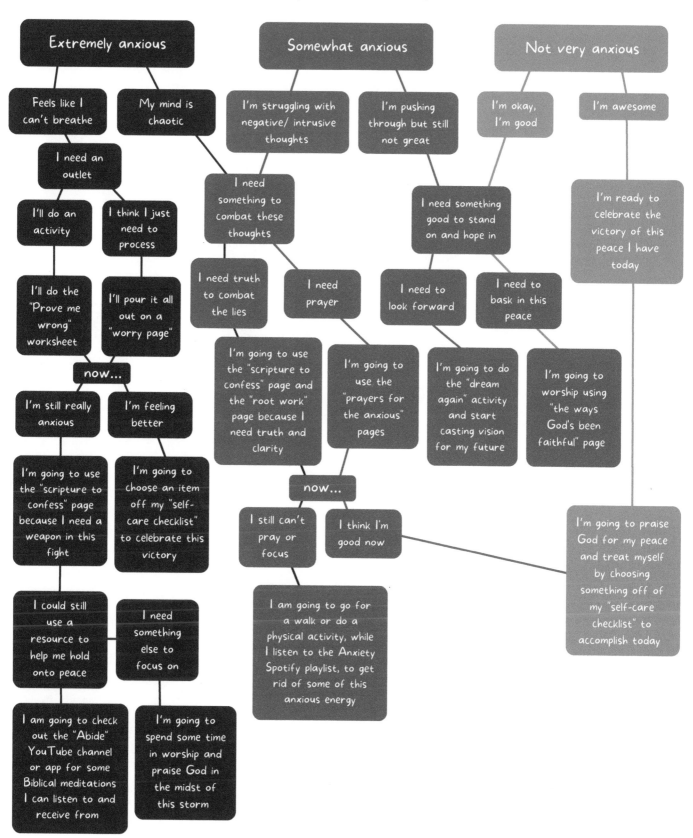

Extremely anxious

- Feels like I can't breathe
  - I need an outlet
    - I'll do an activity
      - I'll do the "Prove me wrong" worksheet
    - I think I just need to process
      - I'll pour it all out on a "worry page"
- My mind is chaotic

now...

- I'm still really anxious
  - I'm going to use the "scripture to confess" page because I need a weapon in this fight
    - I could still use a resource to help me hold onto peace
      - I am going to check out the "Abide" YouTube channel or app for some Biblical meditations I can listen to and receive from
    - I need something else to focus on
      - I'm going to spend some time in worship and praise God in the midst of this storm
- I'm feeling better
  - I'm going to choose an item off my "self-care checklist" to celebrate this victory

Somewhat anxious

- I'm struggling with negative/ intrusive thoughts
  - I need something to combat these thoughts
    - I need truth to combat the lies
      - I'm going to use the "scripture to confess" page and the "root work" page because I need truth and clarity
    - I need prayer
      - I'm going to use the "prayers for the anxious" pages
- I'm pushing through but still not great
  - I need something good to stand on and hope in
    - I need to look forward
      - I'm going to do the "dream again" activity and start casting vision for my future
    - I need to bask in this peace
      - I'm going to worship using "the ways God's been faithful" page

now...

- I still can't pray or focus
  - I am going to go for a walk or do a physical activity, while I listen to the Anxiety Spotify playlist, to get rid of some of this anxious energy
- I think I'm good now

Not very anxious

- I'm okay, I'm good
- I'm awesome
  - I'm ready to celebrate the victory of this peace I have today
    - I'm going to praise God for my peace and treat myself by choosing something off of my "self-care checklist" to accomplish today

Dream again

If you could do or be anything what would that be? Write down your craziest dreams in the space below. The ones you've always been afraid of. The ones that seem impossible; the ones you forgot about but didn't really forget about and dream again. Dream big impossible dreams and remember that you serve a bigger God for whom nothing is impossible.

Prove me wrong

A lot of times we cry out to God for answers but don't give Him the space or the time to actually respond. Take some time to write down your fears and challenge God to prove them wrong. Then listen and wait. Sit in prayer or in worship and listen for His voice. Crack open your Bible and find scriptures that counter those fears and let God minister to you through them. Let Him in and give Him room to respond to your cries. Write down what He said and showed you in the rebuttal column.

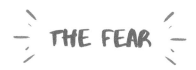 THE FEAR

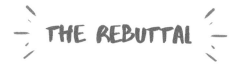 THE REBUTTAL

PROVE ME WRONG

PROVE ME WRONG

PROVE ME WRONG

PROVE ME WRONG

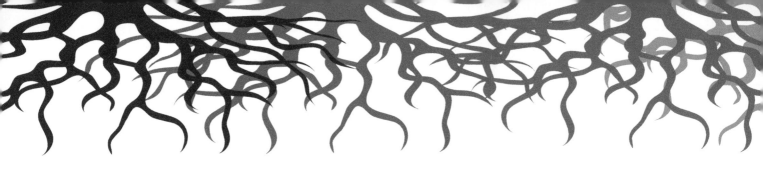

Root work

At the root of every anxious thought is a lie. A lie about you; a lie about God's character towards you; a lie about the world around you and/or the people in it. Fill in the blanks below and practice tracing anxiety back to it's root.

Anxious thought: _____
Represents a fear of _____
Which is really the fear of _____
Which is really the belief that _____
and tells me I am _____
and says God is _____
So this thought, at it's root is just a lie about _____
_____

Anxious thought: _____
Represents a fear of _____
Which is really the fear of _____
Which is really the belief that _____
and tells me I am _____
and says God is _____
So this thought, at it's root is just a lie about _____
_____

Anxious thought: _____
Represents a fear of _____
Which is really the fear of _____
Which is really the belief that _____
and tells me I am _____
and says God is _____
So this thought, at it's root is just a lie about _____
_____

Anxious thought: _____
Represents a fear of _____
Which is really the fear of _____
Which is really the belief that _____
and tells me I am _____
and says God is _____
So this thought, at it's root is just a lie about _____
_____

Anxious thought: _____
Represents a fear of _____
Which is really the fear of _____
Which is really the belief that _____
and tells me I am _____
and says God is _____
So this thought, at it's root is just a lie about _____
_____

Anxious thought: _____
Represents a fear of _____
Which is really the fear of _____
Which is really the belief that _____
and tells me I am _____
and says God is _____
So this thought, at it's root is just a lie about _____
_____

Scripture to confess

Over my future

"No eye has seen, no ear has heard and no mind can know the things God has prepared for me because I love Him. God said that His plans for me are good; that they are plans to give me a future and a hope and I believe that! I believe I will see the goodness of the Lord in the land of the living and that He who began a good work in me will carry it on to completion. His good purpose will always prevail and His will, will be done."

Over my mind

"God has not given me a spirit of fear but of POWER, LOVE and a SOUND MIND. I do not lean on my own understanding but in all my ways acknowledge God. I set my mind on what is true, noble and praise-worthy; things above, not beneath. God knows me; He has seen my thoughts afar off. He tests my anxious thoughts; leading me in the way everlasting. I take every thought captive and submit it to Christ until it shows itself obedient to the knowledge of God or contrary. I demolish every argument and pretense that opposes the truth."

Over difficult situations

"The sufferings of this present time are not even worth comparing with the glory that will be revealed. God is near to me when I'm broken-hearted; He hears my cries and has promised to never leave me nor forsake me. Because I look to Him my face is radiant, and my trust is not misplaced. I will not be put to shame for He is trustworthy. I call this to mind: because of the Lord's great love I am not consumed. For though I am overwhelmed, persecuted and struck down, I will not be abandoned or destroyed. For nothing can pluck me from God's grasp."

Over my body

"Though my flesh and heart may fail, God is the strength of my heart and my portion forever. He brings life to my mortal body through the same Spirit that raised Christ from the dead; resurrection lives in me. My body is a sanctuary for the most high God and by Christ's wounds, I have been healed. Not only is my name written in heaven but I have been given authority over all the powers of the enemy; to tread on serpents and scorpions without harm."

Over the world around me

"The Lord is on my side, I will not be afraid. What can mere mortals do to me for if my God is for me who can stand against me! I can dwell in peace knowing that Christ has overcome the world and through Him, I have been named more than a conqueror. My heritage as a servant of the Lord is this: No weapon formed against me shall prosper and every tongue that rises up against me in judgement will be condemned. And when I intercede on behalf of others, I know God hears me and my prayers are powerful and effective ."

Over my family

"I abide in God and His words abide in me, whatever I ask in His name, in accordance with His will, I know I will receive. Like Moses stood, I stand in the gap for my family, praying for their protection and salvation. Knowing that God is patient, not wanting anyone to perish and for all to come to the knowledge of truth. He is my family's refuge and fortress; He goes before them and won't ever forsake them. His eyes and ears are open and attentive to the prayers made in my house because my house bears His name. We are His chosen, beloved people whom He protects."

Over things I can't change

"The Lord is my strength and shield; in Him my heart trusts. Though I may not understand it, all things work together for my good because I love God and am called according to His purpose. The thief came to steal, kill and destroy, but Jesus came that I might have life and life more abundantly. So, I will not be afraid or discouraged, for the Lord my God is with me wherever I go. He will make my righteous reward like the dawn and my vindication like the noonday. I humble myself under His mighty hand, submitting all my ways to Him, that He may lift me up in due time."

Over things I can change

"As I continually renew my mind in Christ Jesus, I am able to discern what is the good, acceptable and perfect will of God for my life. For He is at work within me, helping me desire and act on behalf of His good purpose. It is no longer I who live but Christ who lives in me, who empowers me to live according to my faith, not my flesh. To call things that aren't yet as though they were; to speak life over myself and others; to live not by what I see but what I believe and hope for, knowing that my hope is not in vain."

Over my sin

"I am no longer a slave to sin; the person I used to be was crucified with Christ. I have been set free from the law of sin and death. The blood of Jesus covers me like a garment so that when the father looks at me, all He sees is the righteous blood of His son. My sins are no more. God's grace is not only sufficient for me, but it is His divine power that gives me everything I need to live a godly life. I despise the shame, just like Jesus did on the cross. I humbly pray and seek God's face, confessing my sins, knowing He is faithful and just, and will forgive and purify me of unrighteousness. ."

Scripture to confess
scripture references

1 Corinthians 2:9	2 Timothy 1:7	Romans 8:18
Jeremiah 29:11	Proverbs 3:5-6	Psalm 34:18
Psalm 27:13	Philippians 4:8	Deuteronomy 31:6
Philippians 1:6	Colossians 3:2	Psalm 34:5
Proverbs 19:21	Psalm 139:1-2	Lamentations 3:21-24
	Psalm 139:23-24	2 Corinthians 4:8-9
	2 Corinthians 10:5	John 10:28

Psalm 73:26	Psalm 118:6	John 15:7
Romans 6:10-11	Romans 8:31	Psalm 106:23
1 Corinthians 3:16	John 16:33	2 Peter 3:9
Isaiah 53:5	Romans 8:37	1 Timothy 2:1-4
Luke 10:19-20	Isaiah 54:17	Psalm 46:1
	James 5:16	Deuteronomy 31:8
		2 Chronicles 7:15
		.Psalm 100:3

Psalm 28:7	Romans 12:2	Romans 6:6
Romans 8:28	Philippians 2:13	Romans 8:2
John 10:10	Galatians 2:20	Isaiah 61:10
Joshua 1:9	Galatians 5:16	Galatians 3:27
Psalm 37:6	Hebrews 11:1	Isaiah 43:25
1 Peter 5:6	Proverbs 30:32	2 Corinthians 12:9
	2 Corinthians 5:7	2 Peter 1:3
	Romans 5:5	Hebrews 12:2
		2 Chronicles 7:14
		1 John 1:9

Self-care checklist

Taking care of yourself and being a good steward over this temple (your body) mentally, physically and spiritually is not only important but Biblical. You can't love others as yourself if you don't even care for yourself and you definitely can't pour into others when you're empty. So, always keep your heart set on glorifying God in whatever you do but take good care of the love of God's life (aka you). Pick an item from the list whenever you feel the need and fill in the extra numbers with self-care ideas tailored to you.

1. Talk to a good friend
2. Eat a sweet treat
3. Enjoy the weather outside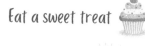
4. Learn a <u>new</u> skill
5. Take a nap
6. Sit back and listen to music or a podcast and do nothing but listen
7. Dance- dance like a maniac just for the fun of it
8. Start reading that book of the Bible you've always been curious about
9. Find a place to sit under the sky and enjoy the clouds or enjoy the stars
10. Take yourself out on a date
11. Laugh- Find something to laugh about (watch a funny movie or comedian, laugh with a friend, read a funny book)

12. Clean/organize something that really needs it
13. Put down the tech for a set period of time and just be
14. Go to a new place you've never been before
15. Do a fun activity/exercise routine
16. Find a quiet space to sit and rest/decompress
17. Do something creative
18. Be a blessing to someone else
19. Say "no" to something you don't want to do
20. Start a project you've been wanting to work on
21. Cook a meal or bake something

22. Give yourself a spa-like experience at home
23. Do something you've been scared to do- Be brave

I am brave

24. Get dressed up nice just because – life is an occasion
25. Spend some time in worship and rest in the presence of God
26.
27.
28.
29.
30.
31.

Prayers for the anxious

When words fail you...

"My words fail me Lord. I don't know how to even begin praying for myself right now but I believe that your Holy Spirit is here and ready to intercede on my behalf when my words fall short. You know my heart Lord and you know what I need before I know I need it. So, I ask that you would meet my needs according to your riches and glory. My physical needs, my emotional needs and my spiritual needs.

Though I sit in darkness, I believe that you are my light and you have not abandoned me. Even when I'm afraid Lord, even when I'm a mess Lord, hold me closely to your chest and remind me that I am loved and that you are here. Show me that you are with me, even now. Speak your promises over me when I can't speak up for myself Lord. Give me words of truth to confess that will crush my enemy and stop him in his tracks.

Let my voice sing your praises and let the worship that pours out of me be like a sweet-smelling perfume that sends every lie and broken spirit running. Speak life over me God, the way you spoke to the storm and told it to cease-- speak to the storm in me.

Show up in this place and push anxiety out of it. Let your light shine in the shadows and expose what doesn't belong here anymore. Open my eyes to the lies and imposters; the pride masquerading as self-esteem; the fear masquerading as awareness; the distractions masquerading as peace. Give me true peace and true confidence in you and give me the words to continually speak truth out loud, over my life.

In Jesus's precious powerful name, Amen."

When you're hurting...

"It hurts so badly Lord. I can't breathe under this weight.

I am overwhelmed beyond my own understanding, and I don't know how to keep going. I don't know how it gets better from here.

What do I do God?

I can't help myself, I can't fix this... but you can.

You call yourself healer for a reason.

You said you'd be near to the broken and hurting, and I'm both.

So, reach for me God, I need you right now.

I need you to flood into my life and surround me. I need everything you've promised. All that peace, hope and joy. All of it, God. I need all of you. I can't do this on my own, I need your strength and wisdom. I don't want to be lost in this, I don't want to be afraid or discouraged but I am God. I'm struggling so much and I can't do this or win this fight without you, I am nothing without you. Please God, step into my situation and restore what the enemy has taken from me. Hear my cry Lord and come to my defense.

Lion of Judah, roar over me and send my enemies fleeing. Show them who you are, show them you are the king above all kings and EVERY knee will bow in your presence. I hear that voice saying "where is your God now", but I refuse to give in so, God make your presence known.

Shake the foundations, rattle the walls as I cry out your name "I AM is my God! I AM is my healer! I AM is my justice-bringer and salvation!" Vindicate me Lord; prove my trust in you righteous. Let what comes next outshine what is behind me and let my life proclaim your glory; for the places where I have been broken, you have made me whole. And the world will take note of the one who was hurting, the one who couldn't breathe as I dance in freedom and sing your praises. Like the lame man who walked and the woman at the well, I will be your glory.

In Jesus's beautiful powerful name, Amen."

Prayers for the anxious

When your mind is chaotic...

"Lord, I come before you today, desperately in need of your help. My mind feels out of control, my thoughts are all over the place and I am struggling to focus on anything other than worry and fear. It's hard for me to access peace right now Lord but I know that you're there. I know that you hear me, and I know that I am not alone in this chaos. So, I am asking you right now to come alongside me and wash me in your peace. Restore my mind to righteous judgment; renew my mind with clarity in you. Search me God, and if there is any darkness, sin or brokenness in me, purify me of it. Help me to focus on the good, on the positive and on the life-giving thoughts that point me towards you. Remind me of your promises and of your truths. Prince of peace, come sit beside me right now and let your presence wash over the chaos assaulting my mind. Sit with me in this place and wrap me in your comforting embrace. Help my mind to become clear and bring vision to my eyes; bring things into focus and help me discern the lies from the truth. In the name of Jesus, I come against every attack of the enemy on my mind and every argument, every lie that has made itself at home in my heart and in my thought patterns. I come against them all right now and I pray that your light would pierce through the shadows and help me to think, dream and imagine in the way you created me to. Lord, help me throw out all of these anxious, intrusive thoughts and focus on you and on who you have said I am. Not on who anxiety and fear are trying to tell me I am right now. Comfort me Lord. and unlock the words that have been sown into the soil of my heart; the truths that you have spoken over me. Help me to find rest in you. I don't know how to truly rest yet Lord but I know you can teach me how and lead me beside still waters. Help me to trust you, even in my disappointment. Help me to draw close to you, even in my fear. Make your heart for me apparent and help me to take courageous steps of faith towards you and the things you have for me. Help me bring these thoughts into obedient submission. In Jesus's name, I place these burdens at your feet and these fears in your hands, Amen."

ways God's been faithful

Done ✓

CPSIA information can be obtained
at www.ICGtesting.com
Printed in the USA
LVHW071345050622
720529LV00008B/93